Revised 20160401

Note.

This book started as out as a series of manuscripts, papers and journal notes, and you will see all three referenced throughout this book.

Neither entitlement or confrontation are intended in this manuscript, however during the development of this manuscript, I was careful to include only survivors or those experiencing the pain and deficits of neurological disorders, and not ask for the feedback of caregivers.

This was done in order that a thorough and honest handling of each subject could be achieved although the down side is the manuscript is one-sided. In every section I hope that you can see our understanding of difficulties that finding solutions will be for both of us and our willingness to work with you, as we ask for your help.

A view from the inside.
Table of Contents.

Contents

A view from the inside.

I have written this to you if:

- You are a survivor, or an individual with long term neurological deficits:

My hope is, as you read this, or have someone read it to you, that you will find new ways to openly express yourself and communicate with your loved ones, caregivers and medical professionals. I hope that as you read and identify with many of the emotions expressed in these pages, that you will be encouraged and empowered through your own personal journey.

- You are someone who cares for, or cares about a survivor or an individual with long term neurological deficits, or someone in the medical community:

In this document, I hope that you will find new and significant ways to understand some things which have been difficult for those you care for to express, and that you will find new ways to connect with them.

Throughout this manuscript, you will notice that the viewpoint jumps from first to third person constantly. This is because I am both writing as one who is trying to study the subject matter, and one is experiencing these issues first-hand. When I say "I" or "us", I am referring to survivors, or those who are experiencing long term effects of injury or disease. When I say "you", I mean family, caregivers, and the medical community at large

Several good short stories have been written from a survivor's point of view, expressing those difficulties in managing what was once the routines of life. With humor and human interest we, as survivors, can identify with the story teller and laugh and cry with them.

Caregivers and the medical community have also written good short stories, many ending with life lessons and instructions on how to care for survivors.

This little book attempts to present a deeper view of the survivor, not just from the glimpse of a story, but from the challenge of a new life.

This manuscript is a personal journey for me, as much as it is a personal journal. From four years of notes since my stroke in 2008, rapid recovery, and sudden regression in 2011, the real impetus for writing this manuscript came about as I started talking to others with neurological problems, discovering how much of their own journey is like my own.

I have also sought to include the thoughts and input of several others with a range of life-altering neurological illnesses such as MS, Limes, TNA, etc., making a distinction that each of these occurred to individuals who had highly engaged mental and social activities, and then had their lives altered because of an accident or illness.

This book does not intend to deal with mental illness, or individuals who have had to cope with mental conditions since birth or from a very young age.

This manuscript does deal with very serious emotional issues, which I have chosen to use this manuscript to openly and transparently discuss. I am confident that these issues are normal and widespread among survivors and those with ongoing neurological deficits and that is why they are needed to be discussed. I am also certain that for that any one of these emotional issues, that most readers have either gone through it, are going through it, or will go through it again. This is why I believe that making the connections between caregivers, family and survivors that I describe in this document is so important.

So please join me, join us, on a view from the inside.

A personal Introduction.

Before 2008 I was a highly active and energetic individual. At work, I was a well-paid IT professional. I was also an assistant pastor, and a religious counselor. With several other families I helped build a small church in central New Jersey. I loved to write, and I loved public speaking. As a hobby, I helped my wife who was a ballroom dance instructor.

That all came to an end, while teaching a ballroom dance class, one week before my 54th birthday, I fell to the floor with what was later diagnosed as stroke caused by a lateral medullary infarct, or vertebral arterial dissection. Although there were initial signs that I was improving during the first 2 years, these improvements quickly regressed and I had to give up driving, working and much of my independence.

 Although I personally have retained my intelligence, I am quite aware that I do not have the coping ability or stamina to regain the roles of professionalism and leadership that I used to enjoy.

Because of my love of writing, in spite of the touch sensitivity pain as I type on the computer or the vision problems of using a computer monitor, I have been determined to complete this little book, because I believe it will be useful to many people.

Humility and Humiliation

The question that seems to impact every survivor is also the prime question around which this book has been has been conceived: Who and what are we now?

This (*our event, brain injury, onset and continuous of neurological deficits*), is a thoroughly humbling experience. We have been humbled by everything we know of what it means to "be a real person". By every definition we can come up with, we have "lost it all".

For many of us, the most crippling thing that we have suffered is not a physical attack to our body, but the crippling attack to our emotional well-being.

- A person needs their pride to continuously find and accept new challenges, new goals, and new risks.
- A person needs their sense of dignity that gives their ability to interact normally in a variety of social and interpersonal settings.
- A person needs their self-respect so that they to provide a support for others to lean on. So that others to count on them and that they can feel needed by others.

- The fact is that a survivor's intellect does remain completely intact. Deficits, pain, medications, etc., become so disruptive, that their ability to have social and personal clarity is hindered. This loss of clarity with full intellect, will daily wash away their pride, dignity and self-respect like waves sweeping away a sand castle.

In this manuscript, many of the pages will be directed at things that are disrupting marriages, and therefore the changes that I am suggesting are those that I believe could improve marriages. But although you, as our spouse, are there for us, it is not our personal entitlement to demand that you make one-sided changes.

Elsewhere in the manuscript, pages will be directed at ideas that improve family or friendship relationships for us, but again, I try to present a fair realization that we, as survivors, are also trying very hard to do our best.

Words or Wounds.

My own background includes 5 years as an assistant pastor in a small Christian church and a pastoral counselor, during which time I worked with grieving people at funerals, deathbeds, hospitals and hospices. I had some training on the right words to be used within various environments, and for the most part, I could see that these words were quite effective for helping hurting people when used at the right moment.

I am very grateful for well-educated counselors and well-meaning friends, but now, as a survivor, experiencing constant pain and vertigo, much of the words that I hear sounds like cliché and platitudes, some from the medical community, others from counselors, spiritual mentors and friends.

The problem with clichés and platitudes, is that it can actually be irritating or insulting when a person is deep in pain.

We (survivors) are constantly finding ourselves overwhelmed by stimulus, pain, anxiety, vertigo, etc. At these moments, we act and react poorly. We are not stupid, we're just overcome. We say cruel things, and act in cruel ways. Intellectually, we're smarter than it, but we find ourselves unable to stop, we know we will have to bear the backlash; the counseling, clichés, discussions and threats. All the while, we knew better, know better and are discouraged that we have excuse and no ability to promise that we will be able to control our broken brain next time.

This is my first recommended MUST LEARN skillset for survivors and caregivers to learn. How are they going to handle these inevitable situations? Discuss together how you will

Breaking the Cycle.

Some important thoughts to consider so that you can work through this problem together:
What are the causes of the survivor reacting poorly? Is it
   a) The subject
   b) The current mental state and fatigue level of the survivor

From the standpoint of the caregiver, do you find that when the survivor enters this mode, that they are
   a) Reacting intellectually
   b) Reacting irrationally

From the standpoint of the survivor, how do you feel when things settle down. (check any that apply)
   a) Embarrassed or small that I reacted in that way
   b) Sorry
   c) Ashamed
   d) Less trusting of myself
   e) Less trusting of my caregiver

Some comments on the possible answers. Most Survivors will answer question #1 as (B). Discuss things when the survivor is not as fatigued. If you answer question #2 (B), then as a caregiver, don't give in and respond in kind.

Some survivors will add "(E) Less trusting of Caregiver". This is likely a response that the survivor does not feel that they can be honest with the caregiver, that the "exchange" was the caregiver's fault.

Old Normal vs New Normal.

Looking in from the outside.
One of the common pieces of advice given to survivors is to embrace what I have heard aptly called "the new normal" which is the acceptance of life as it is *now*, by embracing all the abilities and possibilities that they have.

They are counseled to embrace their current life and to find new purpose and new significance. They are warned that refusing to accept this new life or "new normal", and dwelling on what has been lost; physically, mentally, socially or financially will lead to constant depression.

The most significant danger is that this depression becomes magnified by medications that are designed to fight pain or other symptoms. As this happens, the depression can take on an overwhelming entity of its own and become the central part of this "new normal". So it would seem that the advice to not dwell on the old normal, and embrace the life possibilities of the new normal would be the best counsel for the survivor.

Before I continue, I don't want to devalue all the wonderful therapy that provides opportunities to experience a fulfilling life within the "new normal", nor am I suggesting that these therapies are unappreciated or ineffective.

Looking through our eyes.
The "new normal" includes all the deficits that the we experience - pain, vertigo, reliance on ambulatory devices (canes, walkers, wheelchairs), stumbled speech, confusion, etc. It is our present reality that the we must cope with.

The "old normal", how we were before, might now be months or years in the past. But most of the abilities, activities, pleasures, emotions, and especially thought processes that made up our "old normal" are still a vibrant part of our psyche. There is a constant tension of our "old normal" memories wanting to resurface, and, if possible, to be real again.

Of course, If (or when) we could do those things again, it would be called "healing".

For example, for someone like me, whose vertigo makes it difficult to walk without the help of a cane, I have a longing to experience the joy of running. If my "old normal" ability of running were to be relearned through therapy or time, that would be considered to be a healing.
 The problem is of course, most often in order for the "old normal" experiences to be relearned there will likely be failures and many medical issues to overcome such as pain, vertigo, confusion, etc.

When my failures outnumber my successes, depression sets in and my family and counselors quickly remind me to embrace my new life, rather than dwell what I cannot do anymore.

No Man is an Island.

The old normal creates frustrating sensations of isolation within us. Isolated from our past skills and abilities, we feel hindered from doing what we want to do. Not by anyone, but by our own deficits. For those of us on disability, when someone asks us, "What do you do for a living", we don't have common ground, and we feel isolated from social discussions that we used to actively engage in. Even in family discussions, other family members have active lifestyles, our conversation is limited, and we feel isolated.

Working Together for a Solution.

As I begin to accept my doctor's opinion "permanent and will not improve" as my "new normal", I have learned that I will have to make decisions of what I will do with my dreams and aspirations to ever revive my "old normal" experiences.

There is another opportunity that my discussions with others have opened up, that opens new opportunities for us with our therapists and caregivers.

In addition to focusing on long term goals that benefit and strengthen the "new me", shift some of the focus to finding opportunities where the "old me" can be expressed through fun activities for a short period of time. As long as the deficits (pain, vertigo, speech problems, confusion, ambulatory devices, etc.) will allow, creatively discover anything that can be done to give us visits with the "old me".

These visits or events where the "old normal" is allowed to take control or resurface will likely be brief, just moments at a time. Even so they can provide us a sense of joy and accomplishment.

Family members and counselors could encourage us to remember what some of these were, so that together they can help us by crafting the opportunities to let it happen. We also may need to be reminded, although we already know, that since these are only visits with the "old me", and not healings, that there will always be an end to each "visit".

Therefore, it will be our responsibility to take pleasure in the visit, and be grateful for each visit with the "old me", and with the help of caregivers, we can cultivate the hope for future and similar events.

Here are some ideas from my personal experiences of "old normal" activities and emotions that can lead to these momentary successes:

a. Fluid Motion.

There's a normal excitement on the part of caregivers to think of the great many wonderful "new normal" opportunities that await us: therapy pools, walking, yoga, etc. But what I am suggesting is asking us, encouraging us, to recall meaningful activities of fluid motion from our "old me" and then determine how they might be reproduced or mimicked for short periods of time. This can become more challenging and more rewarding for those whose existing motion is now limited by the need for ambulatory devices.

For me, my wife still takes me ballroom dancing, I cannot balance without her supporting me, and I cannot dance with others, but it is something I really enjoy. Initially, I refused for sell my kayak for 3 years following my initial brain injury, but finally realizing that my balance made it dangerous for me to try, I ended up selling it and all the gear. But very shortly afterwards, I found an organization in my state (CT) that provide sailing to persons with brain injuries in Long Island Sound.

For others, it may be golf, or some other sports that can be replicated or mimicked if at possible, for whatever brief period of time.

b. Forgetting pain.
   i. Forgetting pain does not replace the therapy of reducing pain through medications and other means, rather it is filling the senses with delightful senses that causes us to forget that we are in pain, even for brief moments.
   ii. Laughter: For some, forgetting pain may be as easy as remembering what used to cause joy, laughter, silliness, delight. Working with us to remember and explore those activities that delighted or consumed us so. Then develop environments to help us have periods of time like that again.
   iii. Physical Touch. Perhaps the most significant way to forget pain for a moment is through human touch. It is so easy to for the survivor to see their spouse, family members and closest friends get caught up in treating them with a "patient" mentality that they forget that they are still a husband, wife, mother, father, friend, brother, sister, with critical affection needs that only their touch, or the way that

they used to touch each other, used to provide.

iv. Shouldn't Have to Ask. Spouses and family members often have little insight into the severe emotional unbalance caused by TBI and similar neurological diseases. The often excessive displays of need for affection that is produced by damage to the brain is no more controllable, nor the fault of the survivor than was the injury or disease.

c. Challenging the brain.
  i. There are many excellent new normal brain challenging activities for survivor, software programs, apps, adult coloring books and other activities, but again, I am looking backward, what challenged the brain before the survivor had their incident?
  ii. For me, what used to challenge my brain was writing software programs and mathematical algorithms. Also, I loved creative writing, such as this little book, but did not get much time to do any. Now, I find concentrating on software algorithms impossible and doing simple math such as calculating the tip on a restaurant bill nearly impossible. But, with the help of Dragon Speech and other great software tools, I get a great deal of satisfaction writing even though my eyes and fingers are still uncooperative.
  iii. Challenging the brain can take on many other forms depending on what the "old me" experiences were for each individual. There are many "new normal" activities to challenge the

brain that have been devised by the medical community and caregivers over the years, and these are excellent and appreciated therapies. However, again, I am suggesting discovering with us what we felt challenged our brain, and then helping us to repeat or mimic some of those activities.

d. Feeling loved.
   i. Pain, and the depression caused by pain, are often to greatest obstructions to freely expressing and receiving love. Our "old me" included, hopefully, an environment free of such obstructions. In the "new me", constant pain, etc., can cause us to be excessively emotional, which, although it may be neither negative nor positive in itself, will still damage relationships and prevent good communication

   ii. We are dealing with several love loss issues. These are different for all of us, so I am not presenting them in any order.

      1. What is lovable about me? My family and friends' life and activities now seems a whirlwind happening around me; mentally, I have a hard time keeping up. Even if their life or responsibilities have not really changed, my ability to keep track has. When anyone stops to acknowledge me, I am no longer sure if they are acknowledging me

or the memory of me (before my accident or incident). Because all I can see is how I have been changed, and how often I poorly react to pain or the side effects of medications, I find it hard to believe that I am lovable or even likable, and I need my family and friends' reassurance of what they find lovable and likable about me in my current condition. I need to hear "I love you because...." Or "I like you because...".

2. Why is everyone distancing themselves? This is a normal emotional response to the difficulty that we have sorting through the confusion of our family and caregiver's busy reality. They are coping with life, work, and the added responsibility of caring for us. Among the many things that we are coping with (and possibly the worst) is dependency. Dependency is an awful emotional experience. When we try to internalize these feelings and not show them, we can feel guilty, lost or abandoned. We start to feel that family and friends are finding welcome relief in their moments *away* from us.

3. To be loved is better than to be cared for. When we were in the hospital or rehab centers, we were cared for. Our medical and physical needs were cared for *expertly*. But we longed for a visit from you, our family and friends, because only then were we loved. When we are together, we know that you may

have to do things for us, but we'd rather you do things with us. We'd rather be loved than cared for. Even the medical profession and society have saddled you, our family and friends, with the title of "caregivers". We wish that there might be support groups, books, and classes for the "love-givers" and "affection-providers" that are needed by the survivors and those experiencing the daily pain

e. Feeling valued and needed.
  i. Pain, confusion, being confined to ambulatory devices or other medical devices are inhibitors to the survivor's feeling needed and valued. We are not now, nor ever have been, mentally ill, we are disabled, our psyche is fully functional just was it was the moment before our accident or disease set in. The caregiver's frustration at our inability to get our thoughts out clearly, is nothing compared to our frustration of trying to get them out. Our "old normal" included many ways that we were able to feel value and needed. We could do good deeds for others, or perform special tasks at work that would gain us respect and admiration. However, our "new normal" is that we may sometimes be admired for putting up with our pain and circumstances so well. We still need opportunities for our "old normal". We need to discover specific things that gave us a sense of being needed or feeling valued, and then working with you, recreate the moments and

the emotions. Once again, the objective is for a series of specific, momentary events that can uplift us and allow the "old me" to share some experiences with the "new me"

ii. Husbands will have crushing memories of their "old me" roles around the house. He may have been good at solving conflict in the family, or a handyman around the house, climbed ladders, solved financial problems, brought home the bacon, flexed some muscle, or made sure his wife knew she was loved. For many of us, some or all of that is difficult or beyond our capabilities. The wife may offer all sorts of "new me" experiences for her husband without realizing that she is offering pony rides to a war horse. The war horse will do the pony rides, but the couple should look for ways to help recreate old normal experiences for the husband to enjoy.

iii. Wives will have memories of their "old me" roles also. All of the things that she used to do to make the house a home for her and her husband, she may have also worked outside the home, or ran a home business, or raised the family, been active in community, managed the household finances, etc. Now, feeling set aside, she watches as her husband does all these things instead. The couple should look for ways to enjoy "old normal" experiences.

Fishing for Compassion.

There are the well-meaning words that can cause the deepest wounds, depending on who they come from. Obviously, if they come from complete strangers, mostly we can ignore it, but the closer you are to us, the more that some things will hurt.

My objective is to educate, not to script. Like learning about offensive wording for various groups of people, we can, if you would truly like to know, help you know ways to effectively communicate with us.

Mostly, we don't like to complain, or get caught up into long explanations of how we feel, and sometimes we feel goaded into that conversation, that when we start, we sense that we've gone too far and you want to run away fast. Our other option is to clam up and say nothing and pretend like nothing is happening, but that seems to chase you away just as fast.

Also, it can be mildly insulting when you do not acknowledge the shared knowledge of what we *are* going through, but rather tell us that we look fine.

You can see a broken arm, or a broken leg. But you cannot see a broken brain. But like other parts of the body, the brain can be severely damaged. It is just unseen. It does not heal like a broken arm or leg, and often not at all. The symptoms that we display are very real.

So where can you begin?

- We all crave recognition, <u>but we need it for overcoming</u>.
- If we are talking well at that moment, it is not without effort, and maybe not without pain, help from medication, side effects, etc.
- Whatever it is, we are winning a battle.
- It is for the battle that we are winning and action that we are doing that we crave acknowledgement.
- If someone is walking well with the cane or walker, there is likely pain, medications, side effects, vertigo, etc. but the person is a fighter, and they are winning the battle.

It is difficult to provide examples that would work for any two people, as everyone needs to hear recognition in a different way.

- Personally, I do not like to be compared to others, the abilities of others, or the misfortunes of others, for good or for bad.
- Nor do I like to be compared to myself, or my past. I am fighting in the present with constant attention on the next moment of the battle.
- Recognize the emotional state of where I am at. The fight that I am enduring now.
- If I am losing the battle, and you can see it in my eyes, actions, posture, lack of mobility,

thought, etc., show gentle compassion and encouragement in your words that's it's ok to take a break from the battle, and then encourage me to get back to battle, because you know that I am a fighter.

- If I am winning the battle, don't congratulate me for winning the war, I haven't and I know that I probably won't.

Here is a short compilation of some good do's and don'ts from my conversations with friends going through similar situations and I think they can be quite helpful.

- Don't hover over me.
- Do spend quality time in quantity / give me more attention than the dog or TV.
- Don't tell me "you can't do that".
- Do let me try.
- Don't let me NOT fail.
- Do frequently reassure me with hugs or other physical forms of reassurance.
- Don't me constantly afraid that I'll get hurt.

Is there anything good?

Our lives are now focused around the managing of our pain, other neurological issues, and the side effects of medication. For those of us on full disability, who stay at home, this is the central focus of our day, of which the other events of our day revolve. Is it any wonder then that the stories that we have to tell about our day would include some part of how we managed our pain, overcame a neurological deficit, struggled through a depression? The stories that we want to share will include the funny foibles of stupid things we did, fearless ways we overcame a deficit to accomplish a task, and valiant ways we overcame a depressing thought to get on with life.

But as we tell you about our funny foibles we see that it agitates you because in our story you see our carelessness and the danger that we could have hurt ourselves more seriously. As we see that our stories cause stress and that the response is often not to laugh with us but to have concern, we learn that we cannot share these stories, and communication suffers.

The stories that we hear from others: family members and caregivers, are often much more interesting than our own, they include interacting with many other people in a variety of settings. They include humor, irony, recognition that they have received for a job well done, or how they participated in a meaningful social activity. In hearing those stories, we might be able to remember and vicariously live out some of our own "old normal".

Our daily stories are more often about how we overcame a deficit to accomplish a task, a book we read, an object we created. Either we fail to be expressive, or interesting in our story telling, but too often we get a platitude "that's nice" and a quick move on.

Even when we relate how we valiantly overcame a moment of severe depression by new coping mechanism, which we may thought was very significant to us, we may find ourselves being lectured, corrected, or counseled.

Since discussing depression quickly becomes a forbidden subject that no one wants to listen to, the survivor learns to internalize these feelings which may then progress for many into much more dangerous thoughts of self-harm. I'll have more to say about this under "depression and the forbidden subject".

So when asked, "Is there anything good?", I don't know how to answer. Most of my stories seem good to me, but ironically, the impression it makes on my family and caregivers is often just the opposite. If they are a burden, can they still be good?

Perhaps the worst irony of the limitation of the scope of my own stories is how my stories continue to foster the caregiver mentality which, in most cases, I would rather be loved than to be cared for. When my loved ones and friends continue to hear these stories from me, both them (and unfortunately me) start to believe that these are not stories about what has happened during my day, but they are stories about who I am as a person. There is a slow change of roles from being partners in enjoyment, amusement and affection to having to set protective limits around them.

Coping with Dependency.

As a 57-year old male, my condition has forced me to give up driving, my job, and many other symbols of "independence", I have become dependent on others for my transportation and appointments. Fortunately, I have been able to take my cane and go for many thoughtful walks to consider this subject. I did not find much help on the Internet. Most of the content I found was from the viewpoint of the caregiver.

I'm not saying that any of the views that I am about to express are "right, good or even excusable". I not even saying that they don't merit counseling. What I am saying is that I believe that the painful emotions expressed are common to all survivors and those experiencing long term pain and deficits.

For this section I am writing as a as one person to a significant other, especially spouse to spouse. I am hoping that although I am using all first person speech that you can find highly relative examples for yourself.

Our lives have changed, there is a new normal, simple tasks that we used to take for granted are more difficult, or uncomfortable, or painful or embarrassing. You (the caregiver, support person) are quick to help fill in the gaps and make our life easier (and sometimes your life easier) if we are slowing you down or exasperating you. We know that you are sacrificing much for us. We know we are restricting your freedom of movements, taking time from your own challenges, that you are losing out on other opportunities, and that you are sacrificing other relationships. In short, we are coping with the knowledge that we are hurting you. We know human nature is that you could not imagine doing anything else, that you want to take care of us, and that you know that we would take care of you without even thinking about if the roles were reversed.

But as we cope with the loss of what we could have become if we had not experienced our event, we also now cope with the loss of what you could have become if it not been for our event. Coping with dependency includes this powerful tension between what I need from you, and what my love for you could have wanted for you if this had not happened to me.

We know that our new normal is causing you to cope with a "new normal" now yourself. And that this new normal may be that you are extremely busy and require a lot more of your energy and time to manage work, finances, home and us. Among the many things that we are coping with, the most difficult to describe, and possibly the deepest hurt is that we are coping with dependency on you. There is the obvious caregiver need, for which if necessary, a visiting home nurse could be hired, but there is a darker dependency. We are coping with a dependency with you.

Much of our identity now is wrapped up in our dependency, this is not a healthy state but it is a struggle that is common to all of us. Emotionally, we may be wired to misconstrue any normal amount of non-responsiveness on your part as rejection.

We may not be able to prevent our emotions from running away to this conclusion even though you may try to reassure us.

Our inability to rationally empathize, take perspective, be patient, etc., are all impacted now by not only our neurological deficits, and the accompanying pain, but also by the medications designed to treat these deficits and pain. Because we are not mentally ill, we have a brain injury or neurological deficits, we are intelligent, therefore we are frustrated by our emotions.

It is our pain, or vertigo, or whatever deficit we are experiencing, exasperated by the side effects of medications, that is hindering our ability to emotionally respond to you as our intellect rationalizes that we should. The greater the physical dependency, there will be greater emotional dependency. Physical dependency is easy to resource, as you can see our physical need and respond to it, or hire someone to respond to it. Our emotional dependency requires frequent reassurance of your companionship.

Our emotional dependency exacerbated by life change.

What has happed to me has likely put a strain on our finances. This probably means that you have had to find work, work more hours, find a second job, etc. This probably all took place after a period of time that you dedicated to taking care of me immediately after my incident. If so, I became immediately attached to the idea of always having you there, caring for me, worrying about us, being my friend, companion and caregiver. My damaged neurological systems were *imprinted* with these reassurances of always having you around and now that reality of your schedule has set in, emotional dependency causes me to feel abandoned and rejected. The severity of these emotions can be as great as the feeling of grieving which causes me to think irrationally.

Our emotional dependency exacerbated by role reversals.

Another way that emotional dependency may be hindering my relationships is by role reversals. Not necessarily how I reversed roles with you, but how I perceive my overall value to myself, to you, to others, and to society has been changed. Tasks that I used to accomplish for myself now requires someone else to help me, work alongside me, or accomplish for me. Each time someone does them for me, I become emotionally dependent that will be done again for me. This emotional dependency can erupt into rejection or depression if I cannot find a willing person to help me in the task, or accomplish the task, or I feel that the helper is annoyed or perturbed at my asking. If there is a sense of anxiousness or anger in your response, even if it is only because of the daily stresses that are normal to everyone, I can overreact in depression and rejection.

Depression and the forbidden subject.

My original intention was not to include this section in this manuscript, because this part of the journey is so personal for every one of us, that none of us wishes to ever mention it. Yet to some horrible degree it has been a shared experience, is now a shared experience or will be a shared experience, and as those who care for us and care about us, you need to know that we are fighting this battle alone because we are afraid of the overreaction that our admitting to this emotion would cause.

My entire manuscript has been dedicated to the hope that I can enable survivors and those experiencing long term neurological pain and deficits the ability of being open and transparent to their loved ones, caregivers and medical providers, and conversely, that you can connect with us in more significant and meaningful ways for all of us. Therefore, we must also be ready to acknowledge that "thoughts of suicide" is more of a battle than you can imagine.

I want to give a couple images to hopefully explain the battle.

First.
Imagine that you are a survivor, or a person dealing with long term pain, vertigo, loss of job, identity, etc., and have some level of depression, which is compounded by medications. Your depression is a seesaw. Along, for no apparent reason, rushes in a 500-pound gorilla called "thoughts of suicide" and jumps on your seesaw. Because you are an intelligent, or spiritual person, or someone who deeply cares for your loved ones, you have a 10,000-pound elephant called "reason". The problem is that your elephant lumbers in slowly, doesn't sit well on the seesaw, and often has other things to do. The gorilla on the other hand, is perfectly content to stay right where he is.

Second.
Imagine that you are on a very long drive with your family and have just past the last rest stop for

hundreds of miles. You are suddenly overwhelmed with the need to relieve yourself, however the next rest stop is not for hundreds of miles. As the miles and minutes tick by, the pressure and pain build up. Soon the pain becomes absolutely unbearable. You entertain thoughts of going in your pants. But if you go in your pants how will it affect your family, and your vacation?   You think of the damage it will cause everyone if you allow yourself the relief of going in your pants, but you know it's wrong. So you hold it and hold on, mile after mile, waiting endlessly for the rest stop, that you know will eventually come.

In both examples I hope that I have demonstrated both the significance of the struggle that we face, when we face it, and the resolve not to succumb to it. Because our intellect is intact but our ability to emotionally respond to pressure may be compromised, we understand the pressure that it puts on ourselves and others to admit or suggest these feelings to our caregivers, our counselors or our doctors. The medical community has not designed a treatment for us, or for our caregivers and family members, since the medications that we rely for pain relief are partially the cause of emotional imbalance.

Personally, whenever I have been in this battle, it consumes my thoughts, eventually, somehow, I never really know how, I shake it off, put the elephant back on the seesaw, hope for the rest stop.

What I believe is needed is a fresh look at allowing depression out of the forbidden closets and into open sunlight of discussion. Survivors are afraid to talk about severe depression because:

- Intellectually, they cannot believe that they have fallen into this level of depression, they want to beat themselves
- Family members and caregivers have no training on what to do when the subject comes up.
- Our social groups offer silly clichés on how to overcome it
- The medical community may hospitalize us and remove our freedoms

Personal, I went through all four as stages, one through four, and there are probably other reasons that I left off. The surprising solution, when I finally did admit to it, was that a significant part of amygdala was damaged, and I without medication, I did not "stand a chance" or beating the emotional game. Once I started the mild treatment, I was completely cured of "suicidal thoughts".

There needs to be a way to get depression out of our emotions, into our intellect, and into open discussion with our loved ones, caregivers, and counselors, where the depression can be fully vetted, fully described. Because depression will act like a virus and mutate, it will need to be frequently vetted and described. Remember that we are intelligent, so help us find our solutions to our depression through our intellect, as we vet and describe exactly what the depression is at the time it is.

Depression will have both guilt and blame. Guilt for self and blame for others. This is where your patience, not guidance is most crucial.

There is another serious critical need, and this for our burned out close family members who are caregivers. Our caregivers are not equipped to listen to our emotional needs, they have emotional needs of their own, and in many cases, we should be in equally giving and supporting relationships with them. Many of us cannot talk, or can no longer talk to our closest family members who provide our support, because we can see the damage that we have already done to them.

Depression drives a serious wedge into family dynamics, and how to approach discussions that speak the emotional needs of us and our caregivers is a challenge that I would like to see the medical and counseling community take up.

Coming back to the outside - Some Conclusions.

The purpose of the manuscript has not been to script your responses to us. Neither has it been to excuse many of our feelings. It has not been my desire to offend anyone in this document, however, my singular purpose has been to provide practical examples to connect the caregiver/provider to survivor/individual through open and transparent discussions, that will help you help us navigate the journey that we must take together. I have tried to recognize that the survivors/individuals have a responsibility to utilize their own intellect to aid in their care and work with their caregivers and providers, but at the same time I have tried not to oversimplify the direct challenges to the intellectual approach. I believe that there is a huge challenge to the counseling and medical community to develop practical tools to help caregivers listen without burning out and provide caregivers far more support than they have now. I have used the assistance of others with neurological disorders to review and edit and hopefully maintain the confidence that the emotions expressed are common even if, for many, they have been suppressed. I hope I have been successful, as in the success of this manuscript I can reaffirm some of my personal "old normal" experiences.

I also want to explain that this manuscript concluded at was to the be turning point in my most depressive state, from which by God's grace I am well passed now. I only released my manuscript two years later as a book at the prompting of some friends who felt that other could still be helped by my experiences and my writings.

I have written about my way out in my next book, "Building a New Me: Search for Spiritual Meaning after Brain Injury and Stroke"

Essays

Essay on the loss of Pride.

To me, to be a man, and I can see it in most women, so I am sure that it is not just a male or hormonal issue, there is a place for "pride" in your life. Let me begin by describing what I am not talking about.

I am not talking about pride that is arrogance, having the need to belittle someone or some group of individuals because of your standards. I am not talking about boasting, which is the need to make yourself the center of attention because you believe that no one else has a story worth telling, or has a life worth living. I am not talking about self-aggrandizement, meaning to exaggerate your own importance or power so that others take notice of you and no one else. No, all these definitions, I would use the term "Proud".

When I say "Pride", I mean having a personal need to start and finish well, to be an inspiration and an example. To have a desire to face a challenge, the capacity to accept the challenge, the endurance to outlast the challenge, and the fortitude to experience the victory over the challenge. Whether that challenge is an extra hour of overtime, a special team project, going the extra mile for a happy customer, or just scheduling and spending time with the family. Pride in what we do, and who we are will drive us to do more and be more.

For us, survivors and those with long term neurological deficits, we are usually offered "consolation" in exchange for "pride". Because our pain or deficits obstruct us, we face daily reminders that it is often difficult to start or finish well, and although we may be an inspiration or an example to other survivors or friends in our support groups, we are no longer inspirations or examples in the important ways that we used to be to our loved ones, spouses, children, close friends. We don't have new challenges to face, so we are given small challenges as consolations. I don't have the balance to go out and thoroughly wash and clean the car and make it sparkle for my wife, making it look showroom fresh, so I am given the consolation challenge of wiping the dishes. I am unable to work, so I don't have the interaction of teams of people and projects and timelines that create healthy stress and challenge. I have instead about 20 minutes every 5 or 6 hours that I can productively spend in front of the computer working on this manuscript.

This loss of pride in our lives, and our frustration, sometimes even our combativeness to not lose it forever, is one of the three central humbling experiences that cripple our emotions, make us question our value, and doubt the goodness of all the good that is in our lives.

Essay on the Loss of Dignity

Dignity, as I will use the term, is quite different from pride, in that pride is an energy that propels us, while dignity, in my use of the term, is an energy that propels us to engage in social and interpersonal settings. I shall attempt to better explain this concept. One way to look at the subject is to understand how we are normally engaged in social and interpersonal settings, and that is normally, through our roles and identities. We engage ourselves with other individuals in various settings by announcing or describing our roles or identity. Therefore, we may be an accountant, salesman, neurologist, counselor, psychologist, homemaker, IT professional, pastor, dance instructor, etc. All these roles pique an interest in others that we will likely have interesting and amusing stories to tell about our professions, and as our stories and lives gain interest by others, we feel a sense of personal dignity in what we do and what we are doing. Our lives matter, people are interested. We are interesting, we are making a difference. Our acceptance based on two critical needs: 1) who we are and 2) what we have done for others, provides us a level of dignity that propels to engage even more in social and interpersonal settings. This then extends to other settings and groups where we may have less in common, or even feel slightly out of place. A highly respected neurologist may feel oddly out of place by the excitement of a smash-up derby, yet he has his identity and dignity and can enjoy the evening without sacrificing who he is.

For us, as survivors, and those now experiencing long term neurological deficits, it was likely not too long ago that we had several roles and identities that we have had to surrender. In the business world, we had our careers, which for many of us we can no longer perform. Beyond career, we had roles as highly active men and women, husbands and wives, brothers and sisters, friends. We were volunteers, activists, the first to help organize an event, and last to leave after clean up. In our career, we were respected, we knew how to get things done, and we knew how to improve the system.

Now, all that stability and engagement has been pulled out from underneath us. In social settings when the opportunity comes to talk about me, (and I am not in my support group), I struggle, because invariably any story about me, including about my past, will lead back to my current deficits and disability, and the overwhelming sense that I don't have any worthwhile ground as others in the group that I am in.

Each of us is trying to rediscover who we are again. To find a role or title that will give us some dignity, so that we can gain acceptance on both critical needs: 1) who we are, 2) what we have done for others. Until we find our acceptance based on both those needs, the loss of dignity remains of the three humbling losses that attacks our definition of personhood.

Essay on the Loss on Self Respect

In my usage of self-respect, I used "self-respect" to mean the ability to look at one's self with the primary goal being the desire to support others and to be needed and trusted by others for support.

A counselor who is knowledgeable and speaks well amongst his or her peers has great dignity. A counselor who has patients that trust him and put their lives in their care and tell them how grateful they are for their expertise, has great self-respect.

A man who is highly engaged in the office, takes part in projects, and sees them through to successful completion so that his team is recognized and the company profits has great dignity. The man who comes home later that night, and becomes caring husband, playful daddy, dedicating his ears, eyes and thoughts to his family's needs and wants has great self-respect.

The friend who can be counted on to help out, whether it is as big as moving furniture, or just to sit and listen, these are things that generate self-respect.

There are two aspects, first, is the active goal; to proactively present oneself as someone willing to help and support someone else. This may be as a professional, community volunteer, or simply taking notice of what is happening around you. Second is the passive goal, a passive desire to be needed and trusted. We all have a powerful desire to be needed, and if we do not feel needed, we can then take action and show how valuable we are, and how needed we are, and create the need for us. In other words, we can usually "sell ourselves".

As a survivor or someone experiencing long term neurological pain and deficits, the loss of self-respect came very suddenly. We are no longer needed, rather we are the needful ones. We cannot do for someone else, we can barely do for ourselves. The long term neurological pain and deficits seems to attack our constant desire to regain self-respect by doing things again for others. We look for ways to help out, to make a difference, only to have pain immobilize us for a few days and block us from commitments that we had made. We try to make ourselves needed by our family, but there is often a hovering level of protection that we cannot find real self-respect in what we do.

Like pony rides to a war horse, we are told we are needed, yet the disconnect between what we are intellectually capable of and what we have been emotionally assigned to are painful and depressing.

Loss of self-respect remains one of the three humbling losses that attacks our definition of personhood.

Essay on "Why are you still here"?

What is it about you that makes you hang onto me? I guess part of the answer could be found in the human spirit itself, for if our roles were reversed, I am certain that I could never leave you, and you would probably be asking me this question.

For my essay, I have chosen the help of the song "Where Do We Go From Here" from "Evita" by Madonna. There are several important questions that are asked from the heart that I believe contain some of all the questions that we, as survivors and those dealing with long term pain and neurological deficits wrestle with as we continue on our journey, and several significant statements that I also believe define us well. Although I have always been a believer that you should never give a problem unless you provide at least one solution, I am unable to come up with any answers to the questions that I will be asking in this section. In this section, I can only, hopefully, at best generate dialog, or at least demonstrate where there might be a need for the assistance of professional counselors.

First, I want to look at two observations:
This isn't where we intended to be.

Deep in my heart I'm concealing things that I'm longing to say, frightened you'll slip away.

The questions asked in the song are:
Why are you at my side?
Where do we go from here?
How can I be any use to you now?
What do we do for our dream to survive?
How do we keep all our passions alive as we used to do?

Not what I Intended.

This is not where we intended to be, this is not where I intended us to be. Throughout our adult life we have been advised to make plans, budgets, goals, to have a statement of where we see ourselves 5 years from now, 10 years from now, etc., to make plans for retirement, etc. Even in the most cavalier or "devil-may-care" attitudes we expected that we would enjoy many healthy happy years. But most of the time, we took responsibility seriously, we did make plans, had goals, had ideas for how we would transition between stages of life. I have been fortunate in that I have a committed life-long spouse, and we could think about those stages in terms of togetherness. After my career, I intended to consult, to teach, and to volunteer. I intended to earn an income and to give my time freely. I intended to spend a lot more time with my spouse.

Wish I could Conceal what I'm feeling.

But now, much of what I have to talk about is limited to my daily pain. Because you care about me, your first question is "how are you feeling". I don't want to give any answer other than "I'm OK", because some very special aspect of our relationship is fading. Because I slip up and talk about my pain or my deficits, or problems, I have seen our relationship change from lovers and friends to caregiver/patient. I wish I could better conceal this so we could get back to a normal life.

Why are you by my side?

This is the first of five questions. It is an obvious and rhetorical question, but it lays the emotional groundwork for the other four questions. The obvious answer is "because I am!". If our situations were reversed, I would be by your side, there is no doubt in my mind. That is just the way it is. There are dozens of other obvious answers, mostly centered around love, commitment, family, and "where else would I go"? Like Ruth to Naomi, "wither thou goest, I shall go" when they think about us as individuals making up an unit. It is how we model our unique brand of commitment and love to each other and to the world. This dynamic was supposed to gracefully mature as we grew older. Now, suddenly, the dynamic is thrown into disarray, there is an imbalance as my weakness robs your strength. My pain, confusion, and deficits hinder my part of the dynamic. Our "presence" in social settings is odd and different, since there are some obvious "care-giving" actions that will be evident.   Our dream then, that we must somehow protect, is at the very core called "us". It is an "us" that is not the medical "us", but the "us" beforehand. How we protect it, is the challenge that we face.

How do we keep all our passions alive as we used to do?

This final question is in many ways the final painful, evolution of our relationship. It is the transition of our relationship from lovers and friends to caregiver and patient. Everything that I have read on the internet, every article in every magazine seems to point to this eventuality with such certainty that there are no other possibilities, no other options or roads. Yet, I am quite certain that my statement "to be loved is better than to be cared for" stands firm. Because to make the transition, to make the choice of how your limited time and energies will be spent, (you only have so much time and energy yourself), to believe that love is shown best not by affection and passion, but through care and compassion, you will leave us to deep depression.

Any counselor, nurse, medical professional, can provide us with care and compassion. They have been trained to provide these rather well. Only you can provide us affection and passion, in whatever role you play in our life. Whether it is the role of spouse, family member, or friend, we can have and maintain relationships together that will never be approximated by care or compassion.

Essay on the 500 lb Gorilla

I was asked to write more about the gorilla, which is the metaphor that I used to describe the sudden waves of despair that seem to attack our depression without warning. The two things that are most striking about this are 1) so many of us live with depression as the constant or norm, and 2) that the depression is usually held in check or balance, not through medications, but through force of our will, our intellect or our social desires.

There are several reasons that depression has become the constant or norm for us.

The first reason is the stress between our completely intact will, intellect, psyche and the damaged neurological systems that creates a cacophony of deficits. Every morning we wake up with all the possibilities of what we could accomplish, or what we would like to do, but then quickly we encounter a list of activities that our brain says it will not perform for us, whether it be reading, walking, standing, talking, seeing without seeing double, etc. Then as we adapt to the list that our brain says it will not perform, we receive pain signals that add to the list of activities that we will be limited in for the day. Next as we adapt to these two lists, we encounter our social groups (family, care groups, etc), who add to that lists of activities that are too dangerous, or out of bounds for us to perform, or we are not trusted in, or we need to be reminded of specific instructions of how to perform. With each list, our self worth, our feeling of independence, sense of personhood is assaulted. It's depressing.

The second reason the depression is the norm is our loss of roles and identities. For those of us on disability, or unable to work, or unable to pursue their former careers, there is a significant loss of identity, and the inability to respond to the question "what do you do for a living?". Many of us have had to become "idled" while other family members become more engaged in work, earning income, careers, receiving recognition for their efforts, and are able to share interesting stories from their interactions of the day. Although no one is abandoning us, there is a sense of abandonment and isolation as others enjoy the rich life that we are now isolated from.

The third reason for depression is, and I described this concern in many other sections of this manuscript, the seemingly unstoppable evolution of close loved ones from lovers and friends to caregivers. Where physical needs are more visible, you can see someone who is in pain and give them medication, or make them comfortable; emotional needs are much less obvious. How do you know how much affection or attention is enough? Is 5 seconds enough a day to make another person happy? Is 5 minutes, 50 Minutes? How much time would you be willing to give to make someone happy? In the section "forgetting pain", I discussed that there are pain relievers, and there are "ways to forget pain". This applies to depression also. Affection, time together, and attention, are ways to help a person forget pain and forget the depression caused by reasons 1 and 2.

But, unfortunately, for most of us, all 3 causes of depression will be with us every day. So how do we balance this depression? I used the metaphor of a seesaw, which is our emotions. It is balanced by the weight of depression we feel on one side, and our personal resolve, our will, our intellect and love for others on the other side. Because the weight of the depression is a constant on one side, the seesaw is now named "depression", and we can never let up our guard of constant resolve on the other side.

So then along comes the 500 lb gorilla.

It may begin in the form of a harsh word or look, or an action that I took to mean that I wasn't important to you, or withdrawal of your time. It may have been a dream, or too much time alone and away from your companionship or all companionship. But suddenly, without warning, my seesaw called depression is stomped on by all the ferociousness of an angry gorilla. That gorilla has several tattoos, "thoughts of suicides", "thoughts of running away", "complete despair", "emotional implosion".

When the gorilla gets a hold of you, you feel like a mangled comic strip character, there is no defending yourself. You're just going to have to outlast the first attack. Your mind floods with whatever thoughts it wanted to flood you with: suicide, running away, despair, emotionally imploding.

The gorilla is skilled at hanging on to your seesaw. It can hang on upside down, from its toes, from any position. You are not going to be able to pry it lose.

Time for your 10,000 lb elephant.

While the gorilla takes a moment to enjoy how badly you have been mangled, you realize that you are going to need something big to balance the seesaw again. Because you are intelligent, or spiritual, or deeply care for your loved ones, you have a 10,000 lb elephant called "reason" that you can drag in for just these occasions. The problem is that the elephant lumbers in quite slowly, doesn't fit the seat of your emotion seesaw at all and therefore does not sit well on your seesaw, and is preoccupied with more important "real and concrete" things to attend to. Therefore, when the elephant thinks that enough time has past, and all is well enough it gets up, without realizing how tenacious and mischievous apes can be.

Apes are Smart.

It seems like, for most of us, the gorilla eventually just takes a break and goes away, and our seesaw goes back into balance. But what happens next is that gorilla finds a new opportunity, another weakness to exploit, another day when we are feeling isolated inside and then he rushes back in and tests how quickly how we get back to our elephant. To the gorilla it's a game to destroy us, to the elephant, it's a silly weakness that we just need to get over, to us it's a metaphor of the battle of our depression.

Brain Injury Alliance of America: Find your State:

Young Stroke Survivors
A group for stroke survivors under the age of... connect to other stroke survivors. Meet others who...

Second Chance Stroke Survivors
This group was created to give a different perspective and raise awareness of stroke survival. I started it the...

TBI/Stroke Survivors/Neurological
Real People, Real Issues No Platitudes Only members post and see. I created group to allow us ENCOURAGE each other. For ourselves and our spouses.

www.ingramcontent.com/pod-product-compliance
Lightning Source LLC
Chambersburg PA
CBHW070843180526
45168CB00002B/948